Living in a Fallen World

DayOne

HELP!

I'VE BEEN DEPLOYED

Roddy Macleod

Consulting Editor: Dr. Jim Winter

First printed 2015

ISBN 978-1-84625-459-8

All Scripture quotations, unless stated otherwise,
are from the English Standard Version.

Published by Day One Publications
Ryelands Road, Leominster, HR6 8NZ
Tel 01568 613 740 Fax 01568 611 473
North America Toll Free 888 329 6630
email—sales@dayone.co.uk
website—www.dayone.co.uk

Printed by Orchard Press Cheltenham Ltd

Contents

Introduction

Deployment can be stressful for both those in the military and their families. Often this stress leads to serious difficulties in marriage and family life—rates of separation are higher in the armed forces than in other walks of life. The horrors of war are very real and it can take time to come to terms with the effect these experiences have upon us.

This booklet has been written to help those who are suffering with such difficulties, whether they are currently serving or have served in the armed forces, and their families. It is my story—an honest, personal story, written to show that there is life after deployment, when even mental illness and problems with drug and alcohol can be resolved. With the help of God, nothing is impossible!

This story unfolds the life of an individual—me—but it could be anyone's story. Many of the issues I have had to deal with are common to all members of the armed forces. Everyone's experience is different, but there are also many similarities. Stress and mental health issues can come in many forms: delusions, nightmares, depression, hallucinations, and a number of other ways.

This booklet looks at my life in the military on a day-to-day basis, giving examples of some of the hardships that I encountered. Military personnel face many temptations, such as drugs, alcohol and immorality; and yielding to these is deemed to be totally acceptable. We cannot, however, live like this without facing the consequences. Many lives have, like mine, spiralled out of control and have led to complete breakdown.

That does not need to be the end, though—as I discovered. With the right kind of treatment people can be given back their lives. There is much help, both medical and practical, for forces personnel these days. The problem is often that the sufferer doesn't come forward to receive the help on offer.

The Lord God Almighty is by far the biggest help I have found for myself and his ways have completely turned my life around. Anyone who is willing to count the cost of being a Christian and who wholeheartedly comes to God can receive his help. He will not turn away anyone who comes to get life. The Bible says,

Though your sins are like scarlet,
they shall be as white as snow.
(Isaiah 1:18)

It doesn't matter what has gone before, how far down we have gone or what we have done; God can and does rescue us for himself and his glory. God is a God of miracles, and often it takes a miracle to turn our lives around. We may feel that all is lost and there can be no getting out of our predicament; but although we may feel helpless and hopeless, God is not. I can wholeheartedly say that God is the friend of sinners and welcomes them! We are all in the same boat, whoever we are, and we need God's help. My story is proof of the amazing fact that he will help and deliver where we can't!

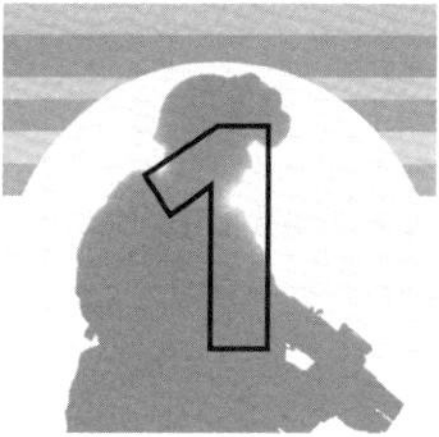

Life in the military

The army is an amazing place for anyone who has a sense of adventure and is willing to work hard. You are accepted as you are and given the opportunity to make something of yourself. Army personnel don't look at your past, as such, in a judging or condemning way. A criminal record, for example, or a poor school record is laid aside and you are given a chance to excel in the training you go through.

I grew up on the Isle of Lewis and had both a criminal record and a very poor school background. I got into trouble as a youth for joyriding and drinking, at that time leading a very rebellious life that dismayed my Christian parents. School was a place I really hated and I did not get on at all well there—my teachers were as glad to see the back of me as I was of them.

Initial training

My father died in the summer of 1985 when I was just nineteen. I think his death was the catalyst for me to grow up a little. I applied to join the army, and after a selection process began training at Scottish Division Depot, Glencorse Barracks. I was keen on travelling and loved television programmes about different parts of the world. When I was going through my training I heard that the Queen's Own Highlanders, my local regiment, were to go abroad; I was thrilled and applied to join them. The basic training itself was very tough: forty-eight recruits started but only twenty-eight finished six months later. On any typical day reveille was at 5 a.m. That meant it was time to get up to clean the rooms and toilets (called 'block jobs'). Dressed and on parade for breakfast at 7.30 a.m., we were marched there and back for 8 a.m. Normally, the section would be standing by their beds for inspection by the platoon sergeant at 8.15 a.m. Our lockers would be open and often the contents—all previously carefully ironed and folded—would be thrown all over the room. There was much shouting and swearing and threatening with the jail if we did not improve. The rest of the day would be filled with physical training, field craft, shooting, drill and much running around. For this six-month course it was pain every day, and the instructors seemed to enjoy inflicting this on us in any way they could. My training corporal or section commander was a very hard man but also very fair, and he would protect us from discipline at times. If we worked for him, he would work for us. At the end of the six months I passed my training and was admitted into the First Battalion the Queen's Own Highlanders, who were based at Fort George near Inverness.

Entering military life is not like starting a job but entering a very challenging and at times difficult way of life. When I joined the regiment I was thrown among a bunch of around five hundred young men, many of them real characters. The lifestyle was 'work hard, play hard', and the powers that be ruled by fear; the jail was where you ended up if you didn't comply. The culture on our part was one of heavy drinking, womanizing and having a ball, as we saw it then. When I first went to a pub on a Sunday it pricked my conscience. I had been brought up in a Christian home and taught not to live like that; but live like that I did. There was little to no Christian input or influence in my life in those years. I really abandoned all I had been taught and threw myself into the lifestyle around me.

The battalion was posted to Kenya for a two-month training exercise. I was thrilled to finally be seeing a different part of the world. The country itself was incredibly beautiful; this was something I had never seen before. We had several training exercises, from jungle warfare to live firing using all the weapons we had been trained on. One night, we were in a place called Don Dall, a hilly, desert-type place. In the middle of the night I was woken from my sleep by a chilling scream close by. Later, I was to discover that a baboon had grabbed the tail end of a sleeping bag with its occupant and dragged it away. The occupant thought it was a lion dragging him away for a late dinner. In his desperation, the soldier tried to unzip the bag, but the zip got stuck and he couldn't get out so he started screaming. There was much hilarity about it the next day and over the days to come; soldiers have a funny sense of humour.

Another evening, I was looking at the night sky in the darkness and marvelling at the beauty of the stars. I was so taken with them that I asked myself whether there really was a God who had made these wonderful lights in the sky.

> *For his invisible attributes, namely, his eternal power and divine nature, have been*

clearly perceived, ever since the creation of the world, in the things that have been made. So they are without excuse.

(Romans 1:20)

These words tell us that the creation cries out that there is a God and we are without excuse! The best I could come up with at the time was, 'I hope so, and I hope he will save me.'

A few days later, while still in Kenya, I heard about the death of a great friend and neighbour at home, a man my age. He was lost off his ship in Australia—news that really shocked me. It made me think of my own mortality, but not in a really deep way.

Trials and temptations

The battalion went from Kenya to Belize and then on to Germany. Drinking, drugs and womanizing were now by far the largest part of my life. My initial policy when I joined the army was not to take drugs at all, because that was the way I lived and thought and worked. One night, however, a fellow soldier persuaded me to try cannabis, which I did; and from that moment on I needed cannabis to enjoy the weekends. Be careful who you have as friends: not everyone is really and truly your friend.

In those days I was very much a man alone in this world—I had no God to turn to. I was a very confident person and I felt little need for anyone else. Life in the military has that effect of building you up: being confident is part of the military way. I thought that I was leading a really full life and enjoying it to the maximum. Interestingly, because of my upbringing, I would still occasionally have thoughts about God. One day, I was walking to the pay office in camp and was reflecting on life. At that time life seemed good: I had all I wanted. I had a beautiful girlfriend and a new motorbike, and my work life was going well. Yet there was a huge void that I now know can only be filled by God. In the heart of every man and woman is an ache for completeness that tries all sorts of ways to satisfy itself—be it through possessions, relationships, money or any other of a million things; but nothing can fill the void except God.

When I look back, I realize that all I had were things that could not satisfy the longing within and that were working together in leading me to a mighty downfall.

Life in Germany was chaotic at the best of times, with all the vices that were available to young men.

One bank holiday weekend, my friends and I had no money. So I took my motorbike to a garage and sold it for around £2,500 (though it was worth a lot more!). I lent some money to my friends and we went to Amsterdam for the weekend. During our time in this infamous Dutch city we indulged in all that was on offer. On the second day, as we were walking along the street, a man pulled out a knife and threatened us with it, demanding 50 Dutch Guilders. We duly handed over the money then ran! He had taken us by surprise, and the drugs and alcohol we had taken didn't help us to think straight. One of our number had been stabbed in a fight before and we decided to return to Germany on the next train.

A typical Friday night would involve going at about 7 p.m. to our bar in camp, where a double shot was sold for 1 Deutschmark, the equivalent of 30 pence. The bar only sold double shots; a litre of wine was £1. Drinking would go on there until about 10 or 11 p.m.; then we would go into Münster town. One of the bars we frequented would be open until 5 a.m.; across the road was another bar called the Breakfast Bar, which would open at 5 a.m. So drinking could go on all night until maybe 10 a.m. the next day; then we would go home for brunch and bed, and do it all again on Saturday night.

There was a real culture of 'who could outdo who' by the most outrageous or crazy things. One weekend, when thankfully I was away on a course in England, my friends were out drinking heavily at the weekend as usual and had gone to a local nightclub which many soldiers frequented. In their wisdom, my friends decided to let off a thunder flash, which is a training device that is really a big banger. There was a bang like a huge explosion and everybody thought a bomb had gone off in the club. At the time, the IRA were bombing and killing soldiers in Germany, so this was taken very seriously and the bomb squad, German antiterrorist police and all sorts of agencies turned up. When they discovered it wasn't a bomb they rounded up all the military personnel and took them in for questioning. The culprits were discovered, but they got off in the end because one went absent without leave and couldn't be found.

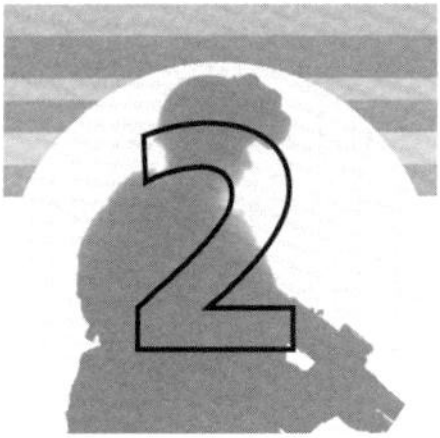

Deployments

Going on deployment is often very challenging in many ways you don't expect. Depending on your job, there is the possibility that you might be sent to a unit where you know hardly anyone. Family and friends are a long way away and communications are difficult. There may be the difficulty of missing wives or children and not being able to contact them for long periods. If there are problems at home it is really hard to perform well in your unit; your home situation is constantly on your mind. On top of that, you rarely get sympathy from your commanders for your difficulties.

Up until now, my life had had a party atmosphere, although we trained hard and worked hard on exercises. One exercise in Germany, Iron Hammer, lasted six weeks when the temperature was –20 degrees Centigrade throughout. Sadly, several young soldiers lost their lives in accidents during this exercise, as almost all troops stationed in Germany were mobilized. When we heard of deaths we always thought that it would be someone else's, never our own. Thoughts of our own mortality were put off until later.

Things escalated in 1990, when we were sent to Belfast to do a four-month operational tour. I was in the Signals Platoon by now and attached to D Company based at Fort Whiterock, West Belfast. Whiterock was a fortress on the side of a hill overlooking the Falls area and Kelly's Corner. When I arrived in Whiterock, I was waiting in the signals store and unpacking my kit, as this was going to be partly my home for the next four months, when suddenly I heard a lot of shouting and a commotion outside. I looked up and saw several people manhandling a person into the armoured ambulance. Just beside our store was the main gate, which had been damaged, so a pig (armoured vehicle) was parked across the gate to prevent someone driving a bomb in. The ambulance was trying to exit the camp but the handbrake on the pig had got stuck; it took several minutes to release it and get the ambulance through the gate and off to hospital. I discovered that, sadly, a young corporal had been accidently shot and fatally wounded by another corporal, his friend, in their room. This was a huge blow to us all and it brought home the seriousness of the situation we were all in. If this was the danger within the camp, what awaited us outside?

Our time in Belfast had not started well and our thoughts were with the corporal's family and the other corporal involved. As the tour went on there were other incidents. For example, a Land Rover was blown up by a rocket-propelled grenade (RPG), but thankfully nobody was killed.

A lovely elderly Christian lady used to come round Whiterock with a trolley containing tracts and Christian literature. She had been knee-capped (shot through the knees) by the IRA a couple of times for her trouble and her love for soldiers. If only I had known then what I know now, I would certainly have made use of this godly Christian lady to pray with and have fellowship with. In reality, at the time, I had no conviction whatever that this lady was a warrior for God bringing the good news of Jesus Christ to us.

Problems with depression

On deployment, things and people get very serious and the pressure is on. Discipline is much firmer and fuses are a lot shorter; life is more demanding, and producing the goods more difficult. The Belfast tour came to an end without further loss of life. However, about twenty-five years later, a young man who had left the military years before committed suicide because he couldn't cope any longer with life following his experiences in Northern Ireland. His case was not exceptional; many ex-soldiers take their own lives as a result of what has happened to them on deployment. When I returned from Belfast, I was very depressed but I could see no reason why I should be. I had survived and, in fact, there was less pressure and danger for me in my job than for a soldier on the streets, as I was working mainly in the operations control centre.

I returned to Germany and this deep depression lingered for a while. I should probably have gone to a doctor, but I didn't know what to say or why I was depressed. Somehow I managed to shake it off after a short time and just get on with life as normal. This return to a sort of normality coincided with the fall of the Berlin Wall in 1989; to celebrate that event I went to the Wall Concert, after which I went home on leave.

Following the Belfast tour I had decided to leave the army and had handed in my paperwork to be discharged into civilian life in a few weeks' time.

During these final few weeks in Germany I was just simply waiting to go home and was looking forward to new things outside the military—but that was all about to change.

On 2 August 1990, the first Gulf War erupted on our TV screens when Saddam Hussein invaded Kuwait. I was called into the office of the regimental sergeant major and asked if I would be willing to volunteer to go to the Gulf War and leave the army at a later date. I thought about it briefly and said 'yes'; something in me wanted to go on and be a soldier.

This was the beginning of the worst part of my life, the start of the deterioration of my mental health. About 120 or so of the battalion were sent to the Royal Regiment of Fusiliers to fill in the gaps in their manpower. I found myself taking on the role of signals personnel for the Regimental Aid Post, and was responsible for providing communications for the medics. On the ground, that meant looking after the communications equipment for about fifteen armoured personnel carriers which were ambulances. At that point, I was a private soldier doing a full corporal's job, and this was difficult. As a private soldier, I was neither getting paid for the job I was doing, nor did I have the authority to tell others what to do. I was glad to be part of the Aid Post, as in my normal job I would have taken many lives with the use of a radio, calling in various weapons like mortars and anti-tank weapons.

As soldiers, there is nothing wrong with taking lives in a legitimate war. The Ten Commandments (Exodus 20) command us not to murder, and soldiers don't murder. Sadly, because of the nature of man, sometimes it is absolutely necessary and right to fight.

We were transported to Saudi Arabia from Germany in December 1990. It was an incredibly lonely place: being not just away from home and at war, but also at a completely new battalion, where I didn't know anybody. We found ourselves in the desert soon after, sometimes static for ages and bored stiff, and sometimes doing manoeuvres to practise the assault to eject the Iraqi forces from Kuwait. There were months of just waiting, and when the ground war finally came it was all over within a hundred hours. The big fear for us was the use of chemical weapons, and at one point we were told to expect 50 per cent casualties.

Although I had with me a New Testament that the army gave us, I didn't even open it once. I thought I might die, and I even thought I might go to hell, but it really made no difference to me. All I wanted to do was get back to Germany and the normal crazy routine. The desert, of course, had nothing to offer in the way of drug dealers or alcohol. The whole time was spent with a craving for cannabis that would not go away. When the ground war did start, we welcomed it, to get it over with and return home.

A strange thing happened right at the start when the battle group were forming into an extended line. That evening, all the armour was lining up in formation in front of the enemy positions in preparation for a dawn attack. I was milling around when I spotted some fellow Queen's Own Highlanders doing the same and I chatted with them. As I was walking away from them, I turned and just prayed, 'May the Lord have mercy on their souls', and I nervously asked for mercy for myself too. I wondered: why not ask for God's protection? But I had said what I had said and left it at that.

In the coming days, all three of these boys lost their lives in an American blue on blue attack (where friendly forces mistakenly attack each other) which completely destroyed their Warrior fighting vehicles. There were nine dead in total, and another eleven with serious injuries. When the reports came through on the radio calling for our assistance we were at first told that there had been a mine strike. I told our driver, who was a Christian, to pray and to try to keep our tracks in the tracks of other vehicles as we were potentially heading into a mined area. However, there were no other tracks. When we arrived, a hasty 'safe area' was set up to deal with those injured and to look after them. After what seemed like an age, helicopters arrived to 'casevac' (medical evacuation) them to the field hospital.

I was asked if I wanted to volunteer to help recover the bodies of those killed; I said I would if they couldn't get anyone else. I have mixed feelings about this now, as, on the one hand, I feel it was my duty, but, on the other, I would still be having nightmares about it today had others not volunteered instead.

Some of the night attacks were spectacular: you could see tracer fire from what seemed like horizon to horizon pouring onto the enemy positions. The hundred hours were soon up and we were left with hundreds if not thousands of prisoners of war. After the surrender, it took some time to get out of the desert and back to Germany, where on our return we had a bit of a party and went on leave. The celebration, however, was only a momentary relief, as once again I found myself incredibly depressed, struggling every day just to get through it.

At the time I knew of no help for dealing with mental problems. There was also the huge stigma of being mentally ill. This is still the case in society as a whole today, although things are improving. In today's army there is far more provision, and such difficulties are more recognized than ever before. I once spoke on this topic to an SAS soldier, who told me that if anyone in the regiment needed help, the military medical services were excellent. He explained that there is no stigma for anyone who comes forward. On the other hand, I have known soldiers to be afraid to use the medical services because they believe it will have an adverse effect on their careers. If mental problems are reported, they are noted on the soldiers' records, and soldiers think that this will affect them negatively. However, it is more important to have the problem dealt with because it won't just go away. It shouldn't have an adverse effect on military prospects; but even if it does, dealing with the matter is far more important. The mental health charity Combat Stress specializes in helping military men and women in this area (see end of booklet for details).

Wives and families

It is incredibly hard for wives and families to cope with their loved ones serving in a combat zone. Wives and children are stuck at home and left to do the worrying and thinking of all the 'what if's that may happen. They have the very real fear that their loved ones will not come back alive. Pre-deployment training takes a long time, so a six-month posting is more like a year away in total. In order to help those at home cope with the stress, the military family is proactive in keeping them updated and informed about all that is going on with their loved ones. Meetings and activities are organized to help those at home get through the difficulties. The families of single soldiers are at a disadvantage as they are scattered all over the country and world. Support for them is limited as they are not in the immediate location of the regimental family or the camp. Many mothers, fathers and siblings have to deal with the deployment alone and apart from the military. The soldiers themselves are having all the thrills and challenges of going on the tour, and their families may find it difficult to understand that their loved ones are actually excited about, and looking forward to going to do, their jobs. Both men and women soldiers are deployed in very dangerous places. There is a Welfare Department within each unit, which is responsible for looking after the dependants back at home. Should the worst happen and a soldier get killed or injured, the Welfare Officer will be the one who delivers the bad news to the loved ones at home.

Loved ones dread that knock at the door that brings such devastating news. At the time of the first Gulf War, our Welfare Officer was known as Captain Terrible. He was a Christian and was able to bring the comfort of the gospel to those he had to visit with the worst news.

Difficulties and trauma come in unexpected ways after a death or injuries. There is the danger of the news getting home to families before the system has had the chance to inform them properly. They may find out through rumours that something bad has happened to their loved ones. These problems are very real in this world of instant communication.

I know of a family in which the husband had been injured very seriously, and his young son was bullied and teased at school because his dad was disabled and in a wheelchair. The son then shunned his dad and blamed him for his misery at school.

However, even if they haven't been injured, soldiers often come back from deployment different people, which can have a bad effect on their families.

When soldiers are away for a long time, dependants may feel useless at home; many women find they cannot cope with the military life and end up leaving their husbands. They may feel they are married to the military and get angry at all that the military life demands.

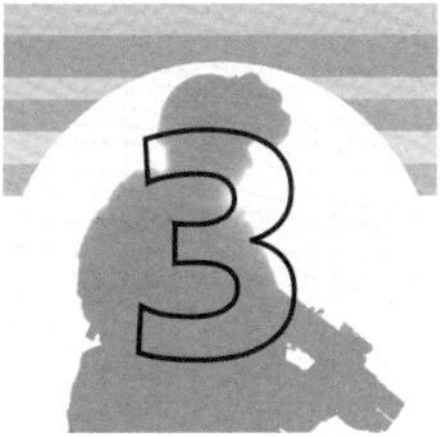

3 Returning to civilian life

Leaving the army is not easy; it can even be quite a daunting experience. In the military, everything is done for you, so it can be hard to get used to doing ordinary daily tasks for yourself. If, for example, you are going on a training exercise to Kenya, you leave your accommodation in the UK, get on a bus that takes you to an airport somewhere, board the plane, fly, get off the plane, get on another bus, and get a bed in new accommodation in Kenya. In all of this you do absolutely nothing in the way of organization: you just follow the leader. So when it comes to civilian life, you don't know how to rent a flat, sign up for unemployment benefit or even manage the bills!

I knew a warrant officer class one who, when he was returning to civilian life after twenty-two years in the army, was very daunted by it. He had a job and a house, and everything was in order, but in himself he was scared to take the step.

When I left the forces, mental health issues were probably being better dealt with by the National Health Service than when I started. Drugs were a big taboo in the forces (though many were using them) so there was no sympathy for anyone caught or admitting to being involved in using drugs. The combination of mental health issues and drug use is not good for entering civilian life. However, God is good, and even if we have these disastrous problems largely controlling our lives, he can and does help and set us free.

I again decided to leave the army. I was starting to get into trouble and just wasn't myself at all. I had been newly promoted, which brought new responsibilities; but in my first week I had been given two weeks' extra duties. This is what happens when you talk back to senior ranks!

I thought along these lines: If I leave the army, all will be well. Then if I get a job, all will be well—and this went on, always looking to the outward, when all the time the problem was within. When home on post-Gulf leave I had a miserable time, feeling a deep depression that was with me constantly. I was going around doing the same old things—pubs and drugs—and I had bought a motorbike. The people I had fallen in with some time before were really not the best company. I had a very good friend who asked me what was wrong with me, but I didn't know what to say. I didn't really know how to express my problems. I couldn't explain why I was depressed or even that I was depressed; I just felt miserable. I stopped going around with the kinds of friends who cared, as it seemed easier to be with people who didn't care; those with me certainly didn't seem to care!

One Sunday as I was walking along the road, I saw several people going to church. I was envious of them and wished I was one of them. My thinking had changed: my lifestyle no longer satisfied me. With hindsight I can see now that not only was I depressed, but my thinking was delusional. I remember being in a pub one night and being convinced that the group on the table beside me were all talking about me. I asked them, but of course they weren't. When an individual is going through this kind of breakdown, what is happening in the imagination seems so real that normal life stops. Whatever is going on in the mind becomes reality; so as far as I was concerned there was nothing wrong with me. Doctors would call this 'lack of insight'!

After some months I managed to leave the army

and I headed back to the Isle of Lewis. I had big plans! However, things didn't turn out as I expected. I was living alone, and when the breakdown really started to kick in, night became day and day, night. I would sleep in the day and be up all night. In the night I would walk around the cliffs in the local area with my mind completely broken and delusional. The main delusion I suffered from was that the end of the world was almost upon us. Simple day-to-day things took on a new significance. For example, when people looked at me I was disturbed by what they might be thinking. This is paranoia: the building up of all sorts of delusions that you think are all leading to a conclusion of some main event that, in reality, only exists in your imagination. Talking to people becomes difficult because the mind is all mixed up and you simply talk in riddles. There is nowhere as lonely, dark and frightening as suffering with mental illness in this way; it is awful. You feel totally helpless and at a loss to know how to get help. Thankfully, a friend and neighbour suggested that I go and see a doctor, and this little pointer really helped. I visited a doctor and told him frankly the way I was thinking; he sent me to a psychiatrist the same day. The psychiatrist prescribed medication and sent me to Glasgow to have a scan to see if there was any disease or damage in my head. The stigma attached was considerable, and most people ridiculed and laughed at me and called me a 'nutter'!

At some point in the midst of this I had started going to church on and off. Sadly, some Christians treated me with scorn and the same ridicule as everyone else. After a little bit of rejigging, the medication I was prescribed started to work and I began to feel better. Every day it was like waking up from a nightmare, and each day I felt increasingly better. It was embarrassing to remember the kinds of things I had been saying, thinking and doing. Nevertheless, I started to enjoy church, but I was still struggling with sin and drugs and various other things that a Christian ought not to do.

After getting better, I stopped taking the medication, which wasn't a good idea as I began to deteriorate again after about six months. I thought that when I got better I wouldn't need the medication any more—and nobody told me anything different.

This process took about five years, and at times I found myself in really dangerous situations. One day, I was standing on a cliff about a hundred feet high with a thought in my head suggesting that if I jumped off, God would catch me. Thankfully, I remembered the commandment not to murder, and looking down

I could see the water breaking over the rocks below—so I walked away.

Another time, when I was employed by the International Committee of the Red Cross, I was on my way to Chechnya in Russia to work as a communications specialist. As I was leaving Lewis to go to Geneva, my mind started to break down again, and by the time I arrived I was in a bad state. I was going to be sent from Geneva to Chechnya in the coming days but my ICRC employer realized that something was wrong; once again I can look back with gratitude to God for preventing me from going into a situation that would have made things worse. I really believe the Lord in his goodness was looking after me in all of these situations; he was with me, although I was struggling to be with him.

Around this time I took communion at my local church, signifying that I saw myself as a Christian and was joining the church as a member. Shortly afterwards, however, I had another, final breakdown that lasted for seven months. Again I received medication and became much better over a short period; by this time I had realized that I really needed the medication (I had 'insight' now!). Spiritually, though, my life was a mess, and instead of returning to God I started to smoke cannabis again. I went on struggling like this for about four years. Despite these struggles I followed the advice of a lovely old aunt, who is now with the Lord, to read my Bible again. She said, 'Read the Bible every day, even if it is only one verse'—so I did; and from that moment I started to go to church regularly. One evening, the preaching spoke powerfully to me. I went home and pleaded with the Lord to have mercy on me and I asked him to show me how real he is. At last I was wholehearted! I didn't really understand why I asked for this, but I knew that God knew. Over the following days the Lord answered my prayer and did show me how real he is—it was a spiritual experience that I can only describe as seeing him who is invisible, inside me. With that, my chains fell off and I was freed! I had been addicted to cannabis for years, but the addiction went away as if I had never smoked it—overnight!

There is no barrier too great for the Lord to be able to reach us and set us free. God is a God of mercy and goodness, and he wants us to be free to be the people he created us to be. Without God we are a distortion; only when he comes into our lives are we truly our real selves. Many people see God in a distorted way as well and blame him for all the suffering and evil in the world. I love the great picture of God given in Psalm 145:

The Lord *is gracious and merciful,*
slow to anger and abounding in steadfast love.
The Lord *is good to all,*
and his mercy is over all that he has made.

(Psalm 145:8–9)

Nowadays, much help is provided to enable ex-soldiers to get access to housing and other essential services. SSAFA (Soldiers', Sailors' and Airmen's Families Association—see the end of this booklet for details) is an organization that helps ex-military personnel to get back up on their feet when they have difficulties. It will help anyone who has served in the forces, even for as little as one day, and for the rest of their lives.

I found SSAFA a huge help when I started to look for work in the offshore oil industry. I got in touch with my local representative, who came and interviewed me. I was able to apply for a grant that would pay for accommodation and two short courses that I needed to do in Aberdeen, in order to obtain the licences I needed to work offshore in my chosen career of communications. All of this happened very quickly and I soon found myself in a position to be applying for the jobs available.

My local council helped me when I applied for housing; being ex-military I was shown preference and went up the waiting list a bit. Nowadays, with the Military Covenant, councils and government agencies are showing more commitment to helping veterans, and some things like housing and NHS services are more readily available than they were in the past.

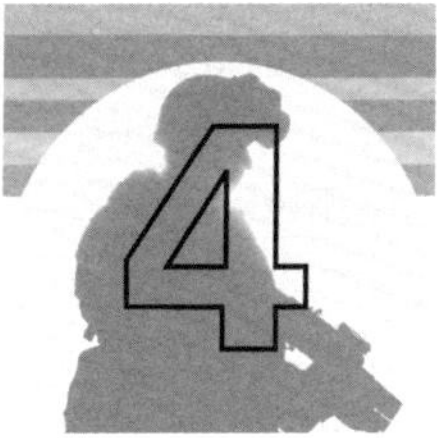

The joy of life in abundance as a soldier of Christ

Many ex-soldiers suffer from mental illness and drug and alcohol issues, ending up homeless. It doesn't have to be this way. There are more agencies than ever before waiting to help ex-military men and women. The main thing, and often the most difficult issue for mentally ill people, is that they need to take their medication. Also, it helps greatly not to take any alcohol or other drugs. I have taken the same regulatory dose of medication since 1995 and have been completely well for all these years.

However, finding the Lord and becoming a Christian has by far been the most healing experience in my life, along with the medication. When saving grace came into my heart, all the destructive problems like drugs were taken away by the miraculous hand of God. This in turn helped me with the illness that had been so debilitating in the day-to-day running of my life. I still take medication and always will; this manages my condition, and in my thinking and emotions I am normal, just like anyone else. But as a Christian, I now have stability in my life; as the Bible teaches, I am free indeed—no drug addiction or anything else enslaves me now, as it did in the past.

> *So if the Son sets you free, you will be free indeed.*
>
> *(John 8:36)*

The next step back to normal life was to get back to work; this too has restorative powers. I had worked on and off for several years throughout my ill-health on the oil rigs, but when I was better I could no longer get the required medical certificate because of my past mental illness. So I went to college and studied IT, which led to a good job working on a local history website.

I found myself increasingly enjoying the Lord and his house and attending all the services possible. There was particular joy in the prayer meeting at my church in Lewis. These delights seemed to grow and grow, leading me to more and more involvement in church life. I was, however, very shy and found it difficult to be in fellowship gatherings in people's homes. Speaking in public was something that terrified me, and praying in public left me shaking. Despite this, I started to feel a longing and deep desire to serve the Lord in a full-time capacity. This may have been selfish at first: I thought that if I served God, I would enjoy more of his fellowship. Over time I started to look into Christian work and felt a calling that I am now certain of. I applied to the Soldiers and Airmen's Scripture Readers Association (SASRA—see end of booklet for contact details) to become a full-time evangelist working with soldiers. The days since I joined SASRA have been the happiest of my life so far and God has done the impossible again by enabling me to speak in public and in many other situations. It is sometimes good and right to be placed outside our comfort zones, as it leads us to depend on the Lord, not on ourselves. I am fully convinced that all I went through in life has been a preparation for serving God now.

SASRA is a Christian mission which has worked with soldiers since 1838 and is fully supported and funded by the Christian public. As a SASRA worker I have the amazing privilege of meeting many soldiers. I find that most young people in the UK today—perhaps as many as 90 per cent—have no idea at all what the Bible teaches. When I speak to soldiers I ask, 'If there is a heaven and a hell, where will you go?' Most reply by saying that they are not bad people, so they will go to heaven. I ask them by what standard they are measuring themselves when they say they are 'not too bad'. I often tell them that to get to heaven by our own goodness, we need to obey all Ten Commandments perfectly: in thought, word and deed for our whole lives, never failing once. As we discuss these issues, they start to realize that this is an impossible standard to keep—but it is God's standard. I then explain that one of the reasons the Ten Commandments were given was to show us how far short we come. I go on to tell them that Jesus came and he obeyed the commandments perfectly as he was God and the only perfect man. As a Christian, I can go to heaven when I die, not because I am good but because Jesus is good. I explain that, on the cross, Jesus paid for all my many failings by suffering in my place, and his perfect obedience is given to me. It is not a matter of being good or bad: we are all bad in varying degrees. It is about what we do with the offer of life that is made to us.

> *The Spirit and the Bride say, 'Come.' And let the one who hears say, 'Come.' And let*

the one who is thirsty come; let the one who desires take the water of life without price.
(Revelation 22:17)

There are no people so good that they can get to heaven by their own goodness; on the other hand, there are no people so bad that they will be turned away if they truly come for life. Soldiers at this point often say that it's not fair that someone really bad can get life, and someone who is 'good' but doesn't believe won't. I explain to them that if two people go to the doctor, one very good and one very bad, and the doctor tells them they both have a terminal illness and they will soon die, but that there is a medicine that will cure it, if the good person says 'no' to the medicine, whose fault is it if he or she dies? On the other hand, if the other person, a very bad person, is in the same position and does take the medicine and live, is that really unfair? God welcomes helpless sinners and gives us life in abundance!

The opportunities for evangelism are huge and there is no shortage of soldiers to speak to. As missionaries, we at SASRA also want to support Christians in the military in any way we can. It can be very difficult being a Christian in the armed forces: you may be the only one in your unit. As Scripture

Readers we pray with such Christians, providing them with reading materials, and put them in touch with other Christians in the forces in whatever part of the world they are. Depending on the area, events can be organized where SASRA members get together and have a week or so of fellowshipping. This sometimes takes place at events like the Keswick Convention or other organized Christian meetings. SASRA may book accommodation and have soldiers come to spend time with fellow believers from the military. At our headquarters in Aldershot we are always happy to receive calls with requests for prayer or any other help that may be required.

God answers prayer

When the Lord answers prayer, he often gives above and beyond what we can ask or think. He certainly did this again with the next part of my life, when he answered a prayer that had been offered daily for eleven years. I was praying that the Lord would give me a wife of his choosing to love and to help me in life. I had spent a few years working for SASRA and my life was getting very lonely; my family and friends were far away. Every day when I prayed this prayer it felt as if the answer was going to come at any moment.

I was introduced to Esther when a colleague of mine, who had met her at the Edinburgh Military Tattoo, connected us on Facebook. Esther was a piper in the Singapore Women's Police Pipe Band and performed at the Tattoo in 2008. When Esther sent me the friend's request I just happened to be online and we started chatting. I very quickly started to like Esther, and I began to ask God if this was his answer to my prayers. I asked God that if Esther was to be the woman I should be with, that I would come across a certain verse of Scripture somewhere to confirm this. As I was praying about this matter intensely, I got up from praying, opened my Bible, and found this verse:

> *Then he said to me, 'This is the word of the LORD to Zerubbabel: Not by might, nor by power, but by my Spirit, says the LORD of hosts.'*
>
> *(Zechariah 4:6)*

I should have taken this as an answer, but I wasn't fully comfortable with it. I was very encouraged, though, and had a fervent burden to pray. On another day, shortly after I had been praying, a friend quoted this same verse to me in conversation. I realized that this was an answer. I was by now fully persuaded, but

I thought that it would be marvellous if God would do something amazing, because that is what God is like. I got in touch with Esther to tell her I would be coming to Singapore to meet her and about the answer to prayer. I explained what had happened and told her about the verse; she then asked which verse it was. I told her; and guess what verse she had had for her daily reading that morning? Not only that, but the verse in question had been going round her mind all the time I had been praying!

We met in Singapore in August 2009 having communicated by Skype for six months. We were married on 4 December 2009, having only actually seen each other in the flesh for a few weeks. Esther is more than I could ever have hoped for—a true blessing. She is a woman with a quiet and gentle spirit and is filled with true godly beauty. Three years after our marriage, on 3 August 2012, our first son, Samuel, was born. Our second son, Timothy, was born on 5 March 2015. They have brought us much joy and gladness.

We live to serve the Lord who has bought us at such awful cost to himself. As a family we work as missionaries among soldiers, bringing the wonderful news that Jesus Christ has paid for all our sins in full. He will give us life and true joy if we come wholeheartedly to him. That doesn't mean that we won't have problems, but it does mean that when we do, he will bring us through to the other side, ultimately to his kingdom in the world to come.

It does not matter what our problems are: Jesus Christ is the answer to them all. If you are struggling with post-deployment issues, you know that life can be tough. You may be suffering in a real and terrible way, either physically or mentally. You may be serving or an ex-member: but Jesus brings light. As with the apostle Paul, your thorn in the flesh may not be removed (2 Corinthians 12:7), but God can give grace to help. Suffering is a part of Christian life that is necessary to mould and make us more like Christ. If we are Christians, Jesus wastes nothing in our experiences: even our trials and tribulations are working together for our good.

And we know that for those who love God
all things work together for good, for those
who are called according to his purpose.
(Romans 8:28)

Nobody wants to suffer and struggle. When we are in difficulty, we want to get out. But in the end, we will be able to say with the psalmist,

It is good for me that I was afflicted,
that I might learn your statutes.
(Psalm 119:71)

When life is comfortable and easy we can quickly become lukewarm, but difficulty keeps us at the throne of God asking for help. God is wonderful and merciful, and he surprises us in wonderful ways in the midst of trouble. So come to him with everything!

If, however, God is not your Father, and Jesus not your Saviour, and the Holy Spirit not your Comforter, they are not far from you. As I look back on my life I cannot understand how I managed before without God. I am also struck at how wonderful it is to know God, and how full of goodness life is; even in the midst of difficulty his Comforter is working that joy, gladness and thankfulness in my heart and soul.

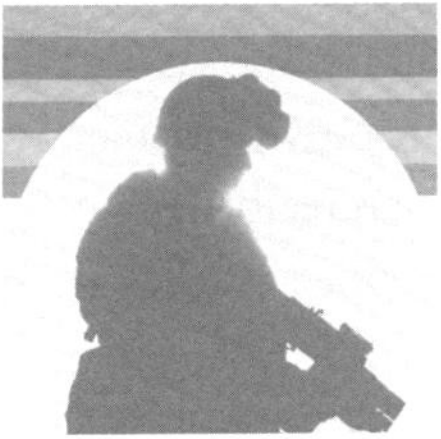

Conclusion

Joining the army—or indeed any of the services—can be a very positive experience and may lead to a very challenging and happy life. Initial training is tough and will test your resolve to the limits. Injury, of course, is the greatest fear during this basic training and can be the decider of continuing or being discharged. There will be many temptations; drinking is a big part of military life and has been the downfall of many. Drugs are a serious issue and the army tests regularly to catch users. If you are caught taking drugs, it will probably mean an automatic discharge.

Being deployed to a war zone is more likely these days, with so much unrest in the world. Young men and women can be damaged on deployment, not just through injuries that are physical but also through those that are mental. But there is life after both physical and mental illness: God is a great healer.

If you are a Christian in the military, life can be lonely and hard. You may often be the only Christian around. Organizations like SASRA can really help to support you in prayer and also in the practicalities of linking you with fellow believers.

Families can be affected badly by their loved ones going on deployment. In some ways, it is more challenging for those who are left at home than for the one being deployed.

Going on to leave the forces later is a huge challenge, but many organizations provide help and support for ex-military personnel. Despite the help, though, ex-military personnel often end up homeless and in serious difficulties due to mental illnesses such as post-traumatic stress disorder. Also, some people still slip through the net.

On the other hand, a past military career can be of huge advantage when looking for work. Many leave the military with very good qualifications and are highly attractive to employers.

Certainly as a person who spent many years without God and going through all of the above, I can wholeheartedly say that life in God's kingdom is more wonderful and fulfilling than anything else I know. It doesn't matter if you are successful or a complete failure: God is there and will welcome you. Our lives may have hit absolute rock bottom, but God can lift us up. We may be in a complete mess with drink, drugs, mental illness and a million other issues, but God can and does set us free. He set me free even though my life was practically over in human terms. Countless others have testified to the goodness of God, and you may know of some.

Life as a Christian is a new beginning, a fresh start that has a conclusion in heaven itself. If we seek God through prayer, reading the Bible, speaking to other Christians and going to church, he will open the door to an invisible world that is as real as the world around us. Being wholehearted is the key to finding God. If you already know God, you are blessed indeed; even if you have gone astray he will welcome you back. Where he has begun the good work he will complete it; and while we disappoint him, he will never disappoint us, but will bring us to a place of perfection to be with him for ever and ever.

> *Then I saw a new heaven and a new earth, for the first heaven and the first earth had passed away, and the sea was no more. And I saw the holy city, new Jerusalem, coming down out of heaven from God, prepared as a bride adorned for her husband. And I heard*

a loud voice from the throne saying, 'Behold, the dwelling place of God is with man. He will dwell with them, and they will be his people, and God himself will be with them as their God. He will wipe away every tear from their eyes, and death shall be no more, neither shall there be mourning, nor crying, nor pain any more, for the former things have passed away.'

(Revelation 21:1–4)

Where can I get further help?

SSAFA, http://www.ssafa.org.uk. The website provides details of the Forcesline Freephone confidential telephone helpline and email service for current and former members of the Armed Forces and their families.

Combat Stress, the veterans' mental health charity, http://www.combatstress.org.uk. See website for details of their 24-hour helpline for the military community and their families.

SASRA, http://www.sasra.org.uk. This organization shares the gospel with members of the armed services who don't know Christ, and offers support to those who do.

Booklets in the *Help!* series include …

HELP! I can't submit to my husband (GLENDA HOTTON)
ISBN 978-1-84625-321-8

HELP! I feel ashamed (SUE NICEWANDER)
ISBN 978-1-84625-320-1

HELP! I have breast cancer (BRENDA FRIELDS)
ISBN 978-1-84625-216-7

HELP! I'm living with terminal illness (REGGIE WEEMS)
ISBN 978-1-84625-319-5

HELP! I've been deployed (RODDY MACLEOD)
ISBN 978-1-84625-459-8

HELP! My baby has died (REGGIE WEEMS)
ISBN 978-1-84625-215-0

HELP! My toddler rules the house (PAUL & KAREN TAUTGES)
ISBN 978-1-84625-221-1

HELP! Someone I love has been abused (JIM NEWHEISER)
ISBN 978-1-84625-222-8

HELP! Someone I love has dementia (JO JOHNSON)
ISBN 978-1-84625-458-1

HELP! Someone I love has depression (JIM WINTER)
ISBN 978-1-84625-460-4

HELP! I HAVE BREAST CANCER

The sense of shock at receiving a diagnosis of breast cancer is real. Once the shock wears off, your mind may explode with questions. Will I need chemotherapy? Am I going to be disfigured by a surgical procedure? Am I going to die? Is God punishing me? This honest account of a battle with breast cancer gently helps you to confront your fears and worries, and points you toward the peace and hope that are found in Jesus Christ.

Brenda Frields has been involved in teaching and discipling women for many years. She and her husband Michael, an obstetrician/gynaecologist, live in Southern California and have three married children and ten grandchildren.

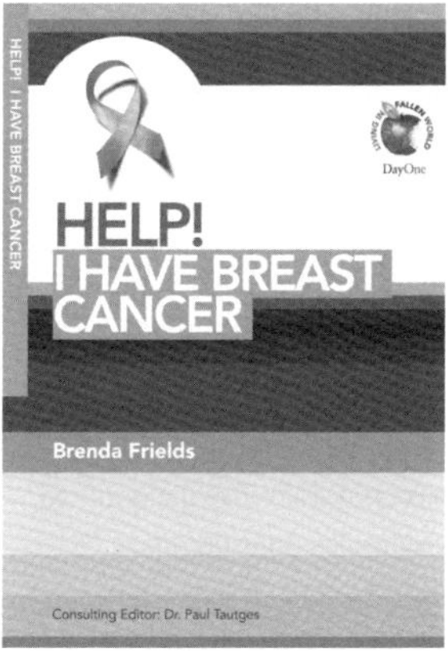

HELP2 ISBN 978-1-84625-216-7

HELP!
MY TODDLER RULES THE HOUSE

We live in a society dominated by child-centred parenting. A typical walk through a shopping mall, or local grocery store, often reveals this sad truth. The almost incessant whining of undisciplined children leads the discerning person to ask, "Just who is in charge anyway?" In this booklet, the seasoned parents of ten children provide frazzled mothers and fathers with practical counsel for bringing order to their homes.

Paul & Karen Tautges are the blessed parents of ten children. Paul is a pastor, biblical counsellor, and author of numerous books on counselling-related issues. Karen is a faithful wife, homemaker, and home-school mother. Together they raise their family in Plymouth, Wisconsin.

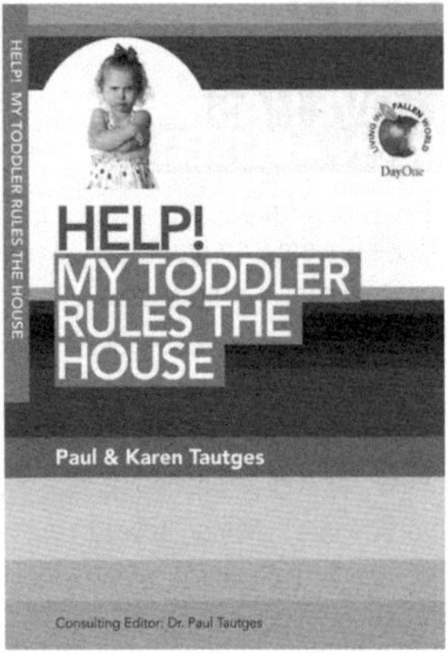

HELP7 ISBN 978-1-84625-221-1

HELP! SOMEONE I LOVE HAS BEEN ABUSED

Abuse is a growing problem, and those who have been abused need help. This booklet equips the reader to offer compassionate biblical counsel to a victim of abuse. As well as providing practical instruction on how to help the victim gain safety and deal with the abuser in a biblical way, it points to the victory possible in Jesus Christ, who was abused for his people, and who has compassion on all hurting people who turn to him.

Jim Newheiser, MA, DMin, Westminster Theological Seminary, has been practising biblical counselling for over twenty years. He is a NANC Fellow, has served as the director of IBCD since 2006, and is a pastor at Grace Bible Church in Escondido, California..

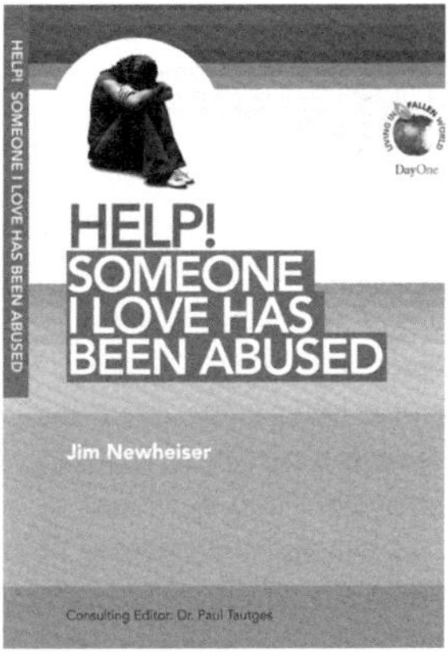

HELP8 ISBN 978-1-84625-222-8

HELP! I AM DEPRESSED

"Life seems so unfair. Why is it so hard? Why doesn't the Lord answer my prayers?" Sometimes the circumstances of our lives overwhelm us and we plunge into depression and despair. Is there a way out? This booklet uses biblical examples to show that even in the midst of great sorrow we can trust God's sovereign purposes, respond in faith, and know peace and even joy.

Carol Trahan (BS, MA) has been a widow and single mother since 1994. She currently serves on the faculty of Harvest Ministries, located on the island of Guam, and is a frequent speaker at ladies' conferences.

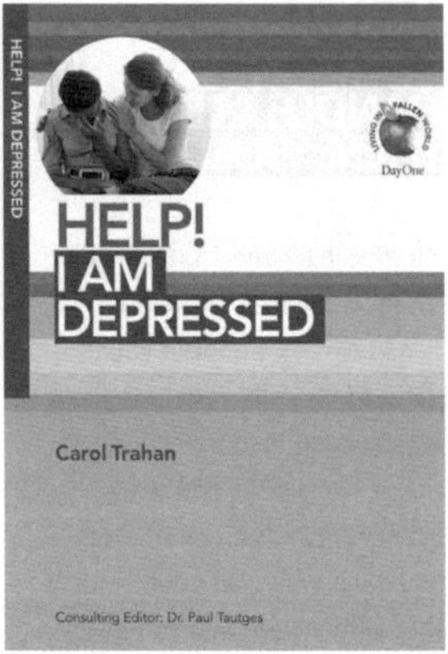

HELP17 ISBN 978-1-84625-318-8

HELP! I CAN'T HANDLE ALL THESE TRIALS

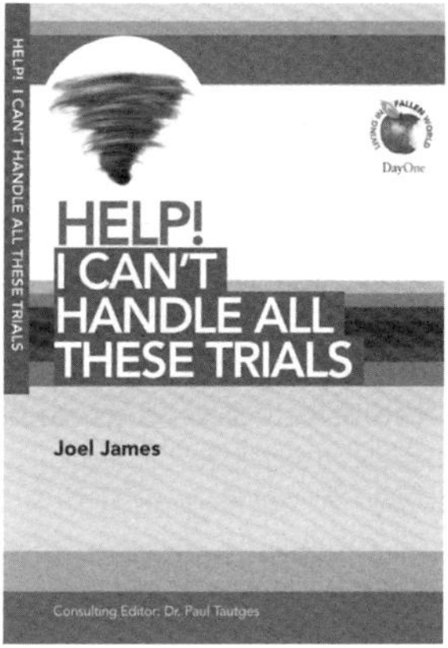

HELP18 ISBN 978-1-84625-324-9

"Who is in control? Why did this happen? What is God doing?" Everyone asks questions like these when faced with intense or prolonged trials. The place to find answers is the Bible. In this booklet, you'll find the answers God gave Job in the book of Job. They will be just what you need to handle your trials with faith, peace, and hope, rather than doubt, confusion, and despair.

Joel James has an M.Div and a D.Min. from The Master's Seminary and is the pastor-teacher of Grace Fellowship in Pretoria, South Africa. He and his wife, Ruth, have been married since 1993 and have two children..

HELP!
I'M LIVING WITH TERMINAL ILLNESS

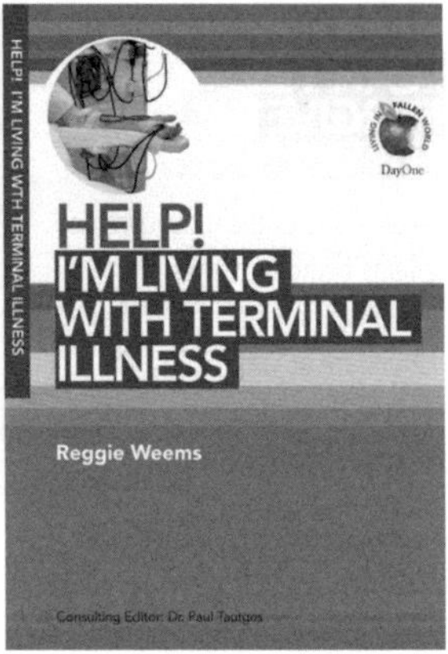

HELP22 ISBN 978-1-84625-319-5

We don't find it easy to face death, and the diagnosis of a terminal illness can be devastating. Yet every life has an expiration date. Written with a pastor's heart for those suffering with a terminal diagnosis and for their family and friends, this booklet conveys practical advice, spiritual consolation, and, most importantly, an eternal hope which the dying process cannot diminish and death cannot extinguish.

Reggie Weems is the pastor of Heritage Baptist Church, Johnson City, TN. He has three Master's degrees from Liberty University and is presently enrolled in DMin and PhD programmes. He and his wife, Teana, have three children and five grandchildren.

HELP! I CAN'T FORGIVE

What is one of the most common refrains heard in homes, relationships, churches, and even our culture at large? "I can't forgive!" The struggle to forgive someone who has wronged us is universal. What is the answer? A fresh look at the gospel! Join the author as he takes you through a five-stop journey toward biblical forgiveness.

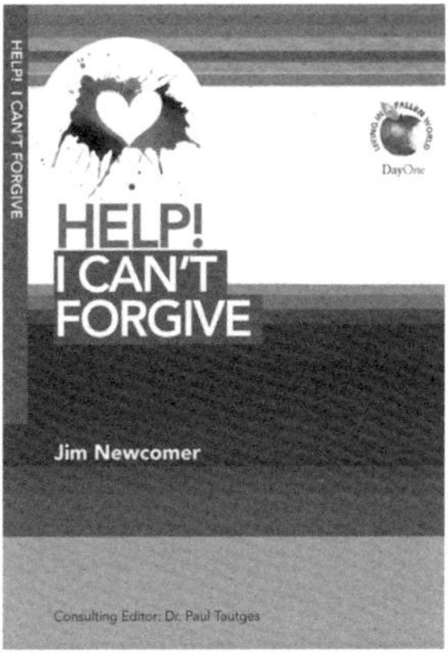

HELP24 ISBN 978-1-84625-325-6

Dr Jim Newcomer (Biblical Counselling Professor, Central Baptist Theological Seminary of Virginia Beach) has enjoyed twenty years of pastoral ministry. He also teaches counselling in several undergraduate and graduate institutions. He and his wife, Lorie, have three children.

HELP!
SOMEONE I LOVE HAS DEMENTIA

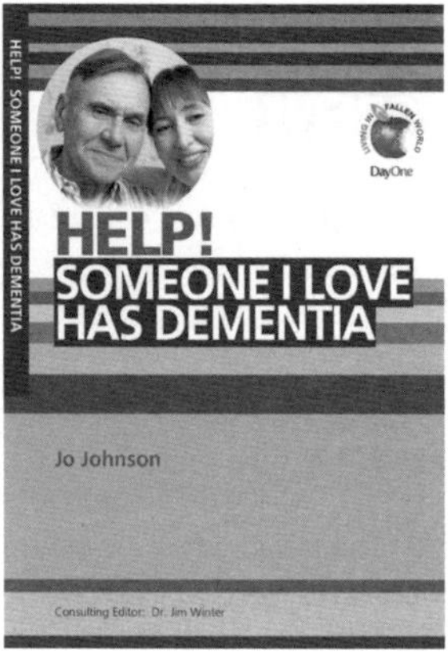

HELP26 ISBN 978-1-84625-458-1

A diagnosis of dementia usually comes as a great shock. Christians are not promised exemption from ill-health or the distress that comes with a difficult diagnosis. This booklet sets out the basic facts about dementia, corrects some common misconceptions and gives practical ideas for supporting loved ones. The booklet ends with a biblical understanding of dementia, offering hope and comfort to the individual as well as family and friends.

Jo Johnson was a clinical psychologist within the NHS for nearly twenty years, but now works as an independent neuropsychologist specializing in dementia, multiple sclerosis and brain injury. Having become a Christian as a teenager, she now attends Storrington Chapel and lives with her husband and four children in West Sussex.